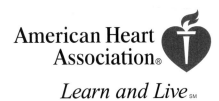

American Heart
Association®

Learn and Live sm

Family & Friends™
First Aid for Children

Provided By:

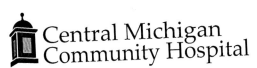

Central Michigan
Community Hospital

HEALTH PROMOTOION SERVICES
1221 South Drive
Mt. Pleasant, MI 48858
989-779-5606

ISBN 0-87493-490-7

Contents

CONTENTS

Considerations for International Readers

The following table is intended for international participants of this program. It is meant to help materials in this program that may be relevant only to those in the United States. For more specific information about your local practices and organizations please contact your instructor.

Page 38	The black widow spider and the brown recluse spider are given as examples of spiders that can inject poison (venom). These spiders are native to the US. Please talk to your instructor about poisonous insects and spiders in your area.
Page 39	The telephone number for the US National Poison Control Center (800-222-1222) is for the US only. Please ask your instructor for the poison control number in your area.

Introduction

Overview

This book gives you first aid basics for children. As you use this book, remember that you don't have to make all the decisions. We will tell you how to get help if you need it.

Who Should Take This Program

We created this program for anyone who wants to learn first aid for children and does not need a course completion card in first aid.

Parts of This Book

This book has the following parts:

- ■ Dealing With Children of Different Ages and Child Safety
- ■ First Aid Basics
- ■ Medical Emergencies
- ■ Injury Emergencies
- ■ Environmental Emergencies

Dealing With Children of Different Ages and Child Safety

How to Deal With Children of Different Ages

Children Don't Always Act Their Age

Children who are sick, hurt, or afraid often do not act their age. Instead, they may act like a younger child. Treat sick, hurt, or frightened children based on how they act, not based on their age.

Use these tips when dealing with children of different ages:

Category	Age	Tips
Infants	Birth to 1 year	• Support the head when you lift or carry an infant less than 4 months of age. • Use a soft, quiet voice and gentle motions around infants. • Keep an infant warm but not overly hot.
Toddlers	1 to 3 years	• Toddlers may not speak well but can often understand what others say. • They may be afraid of adults they do not know. • You may need to give extra comfort when trained help arrives to care for a toddler.
Young Children	4 to 10 years	• Stay calm because they pick up on feelings around them. • Use simple words to explain any emergency and keep them calm. • They can understand simple things you tell them. • They fear being apart from caregivers and friends.
Adolescents	11 to 18 years	• Tell them what you are doing to help them. • Comfort them without talking down to them.
Children With Special Needs	Any age	• Work with healthcare providers to know how to use medical devices or medicines.

Prevention Is Key

Injuries are often thought to be "accidents" that can't be avoided. You can prevent many injuries with simple actions in the home, car, child care center, school, and playground.

Safety at Home

■ Keep emergency numbers (911, poison control, and healthcare providers) near a phone where you keep other important information.

■ Keep children away from things that can hurt them.

Item	Action
Electrical outlets	Cover with protective covers.
Medicine	Store in locked cabinets away from children's reach.
Knives and sharp objects	Keep out of children's reach.
Hot stove tops, burners, and ovens	Use stove guards and keep children away.
Cleaning supplies	Store on high shelves or in locked cabinets.
Stairs	Use stair gates or guards to keep toddlers from climbing or falling.
Guns	Unload and store in a locked cabinet.

■ Install smoke and carbon monoxide detectors.

■ Install window guards.

■ Make sure that the house or apartment number is visible from the street.

> **Do Not**
>
> NEVER shake a baby. Shaking or tossing a baby in the air while playing can cause serious injury.

Car Safety

- Make sure everyone in the car (including the driver) uses seat belts at all times. Infants and young children should be belted in a proper child safety seat.
- Make sure children keep their arms inside the windows.
- Use child safety locks on car doors (if available) when driving young children.
- Keep young children from using power windows and locks.
- Never leave a child alone in a car.
- All children 12 years of age and younger should sit in the back seat.

On the Playground or Sports Field

- Watch young children.
- Make sure children wear closed-toe shoes when playing.
- Make sure children wear the right gear for any sport they are playing.
- Make sure children wear bicycle helmets when riding a bike.
- Check the playground to make sure it is safe and free of harmful trash.

Visit with your child's healthcare provider before the child starts to play a new sport to make sure the child is healthy enough to play.

At a Child Care Facility

Each state has specific safety rules that child care facilities must follow to prevent injuries. Before you enroll your child in a child care facility, visit the facility.

Around Water

- Do not leave a child alone in a bathtub.
- Closely watch all children near pools or other bodies of water. A child might drown even if she knows how to swim.
- Always stay within reach of a child near a body of water.

Reducing the Risk of SIDS

According to the American Academy of Pediatrics, SIDS (sudden infant death syndrome) is the sudden death of an infant under 1 year of age that is not explained by other causes. SIDS is the third leading cause of death in infants in the United States.

When putting an infant down to sleep, remember to lay a healthy infant on his back and NOT on the stomach or side. *Remember:* Place the infant *"back to sleep."* There should be no loose blankets, comforters, toys, or other soft materials in the bed.

First Aid Basics

Being Ready

Overview
It is usually a good idea for families and anyone caring for children to be ready for emergencies and to be able to give first aid.

First Aid Action Plan
A first aid action plan is written and includes

- The emergency response number (usually 911)
- The location of the first aid kit
- Information and instructions, such as
  - Telephone numbers and locations of nearby emergency care facilities
  - Telephone number of the poison control center

Emergency Response Plan
It is important to have an emergency response plan for possible dangers in your area. Have a plan that includes

- How to escape from a home or building
- Where to go in the building in case of an emergency
- How to access emergency medical service

Have regular drills to practice your emergency response plan.

Reasons to Phone for Help
As a general rule, you should phone your emergency response number (or 911) and ask for help whenever

- Someone is seriously ill or hurt
- You are not sure what to do in an emergency

Remember: It is better to phone for help even if you might not need it than not to phone when someone does need help.

How to Phone for Help The following table shows how to phone for help:

If you are	Then you should
Alone	• Yell for help while you start to check the child. • If no one answers and the child does not need first aid right away: — Leave the child for a moment while you phone your emergency response number (or 911). — Get the first aid kit. • Go back to the child.
With others	• Stay with the child. • Send someone else to phone your emergency response number (or 911) and get the first aid kit.

General Principles of First Aid

What First Aid Is First aid is the immediate care you give someone who is sick or injured *before* trained help arrives and takes over.

Safety

Overview The first step in first aid is to make sure you and the sick or injured child are safe before you give first aid.

Scene Safety
- ■ Stop and look at the scene as you go to the child.
- ■ Look out for oncoming traffic. Ask others to direct traffic around the area (Figure 1).
- ■ Before you start giving first aid, make sure you and the child are out of harm's way.
- ■ If the scene is dangerous, move the child to a safer location. (See the section titled "Moving a Child.")

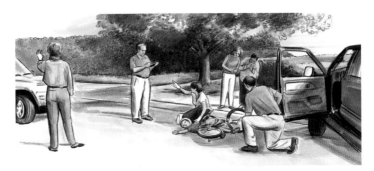

Figure 1. Ask others to direct traffic.

Moving a Child	The only time you should move a badly hurt child is if the scene is unsafe for you or the child or if the child is face down and needs CPR. Examples of unsafe places include a busy street or parking lot; near a fire, smoke, or gas; or in water.
Hand Washing	Hand washing is the most important step in preventing illness.

- Wash your hands after you give first aid so that you don't spread germs.
- Use waterless hand sanitizers if you do not have soap and water near you. Wash your hands with soap and water as soon as you can.

Checking for Injuries and Illnesses

Steps to Find the Problem

Step	Actions
1	When you arrive at the scene, check the scene to be sure it is safe. As you walk toward the child, try to **look for signs of the cause of the problem.**

(continued)

Step	Actions

2	**Tap the child and shout, "Are you OK?"**
	• A victim who "responds" will react in some way.
	   — A child who responds and is awake may be able to answer your questions. Tell the child you are there to help and ask what the problem is.
	   — If a child just moves or moans or groans when you tap him and shout, phone or send someone to phone your emergency response number (or 911) and get the first aid kit.
	• A child who "does not respond" does not move or react in any way when you tap him. Phone or send someone to phone your emergency response number (or 911) and get the first aid kit and AED* if available.

3	**Next, open the airway by tilting the head and lifting the chin (Figure 2) if needed.**
	• If a child responds and is awake, the child is breathing. You will not need to open the airway.
	• If the child does not respond or only moans or groans, you have to open the airway before you can check whether the child is breathing:
	   — Tilt the head by pushing back on the forehead.
	   — Lift the chin by putting your fingers on the bony part of the chin. Do not press the soft parts of the neck or under the chin.
	   — Lift the chin to move the jaw forward.

4	**Check whether the child is breathing.** • Place your ear next to the child's mouth and nose. • **Look** to see whether the chest is moving. • **Listen** for breaths. • **Feel** for breaths on your cheek.
5	**Look for any obvious signs of injury, such as bleeding, broken bones, burns, or bites.**
6	**Look for medical information jewelry.**

*An automated external defibrillator (AED) is a machine with a computer inside that can recognize some heart problems that require a shock and give a shock if needed. You may have access to an AED in some public settings.

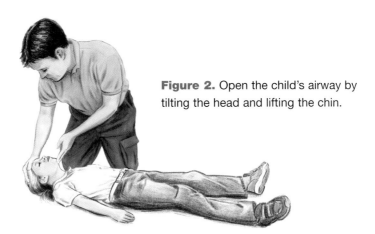

Figure 2. Open the child's airway by tilting the head and lifting the chin.

Medical Emergencies

Breathing Problems

Signs of Breathing Problems

You can tell if someone is having trouble breathing if the person

- Is breathing very fast or very slowly
- Is having trouble with every breath
- Has noisy breathing with a sound or whistle
- Struggles to talk but can't get enough air to do so

Actions for Breathing Problems

If a child has trouble breathing, follow these steps:

Step	Action
1	Do you know if the child has medicine for breathing problems? • If yes, get it and help the child use it. • If no, ask whether the child has medicine and help the child get it and use it.
2	Phone your emergency response number (or 911) if • The child has no medicine • The child does not get better after using the medicine • The child's breathing gets worse, the child has trouble speaking, or the child stops responding

Signs and Actions for Choking

When food or an object such as a toy gets in the airway, it can block the airway. Adults and children can easily choke while eating. Children also can easily choke when playing with small toys.

Choking can be scary. If the block in the airway is severe, you must act quickly to remove the block. If you do, you can help the child breathe.

Use the table below to know whether a child is choking:

If the child	Then the block in the airway is	And you should
• Can make sounds • Can cough loudly	Mild	• Stand by and let the child cough. • If you are worried about the child's breathing, *phone your emergency response number (or 911).*
• Cannot breathe • Cannot talk or make a sound • Cannot cry (younger child) • Has high-pitched, noisy breathing • Has a cough that is very quiet or has no sound • Has bluish lips or skin • Makes the choking sign	Severe	• Act quickly • Follow the steps below

FYI: The Choking Sign

A person who is choking may use the choking sign (holding the neck with one or both hands) (Figure 3).

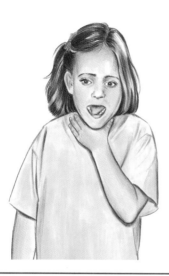

Figure 3. The choking sign. The victim holds her neck with one or both hands.

How to Help a Choking Person Over 1 Year of Age

Follow these steps to help a choking person who is 1 year of age and older:

Step	Action
1	If you think someone is choking, ask, "Are you choking?" If the child nods, tell her you are going to help.
2	Kneel or stand firmly behind her and wrap your arms around her so that your hands are in front.
3	Make a fist with one hand.
4	Put the thumb side of your fist slightly above the belly button and well below the breastbone.
5	Grasp the fist with your other hand and give quick upward thrusts into her belly (Figure 4).
6	Give thrusts until the object is forced out and she can breathe, cough, or speak, or until she stops responding.

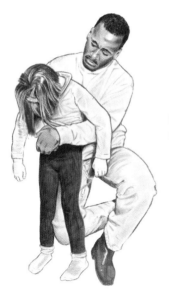

Figure 4. Give quick upward thrusts into the child's belly.

Actions for a Choking Person Who Stops Responding

If you cannot remove the object, the victim will stop responding. When the victim stops responding, follow these steps:

Step	Action
1	Yell for help. If someone comes, send that person to phone your emergency response number (or 911).
2	Lower the victim to the ground, face up. • If you are alone with the adult victim, phone your emergency response number (or 911) and get the AED. Then return to the victim and start the steps of CPR if you know how. Remember to look in the victim's mouth and remove any object you see before giving breaths. If you don't know CPR, the dispatcher can tell you what to do. • If you are alone with the child victim, start the steps of CPR if you know how. Remember to look in the victim's mouth and remove any object you see before giving breaths. If you don't know CPR, the dispatcher can tell you what to do.
3	Continue CPR until the child starts to move or trained help takes over.

FYI: Asking a Victim About Choking

Sometimes a victim is too young to answer your question or cannot answer your question for some other reason.

If the adult or child victim does not respond or cannot answer and you think the victim is choking, give thrusts until the object is forced out and the victim can breathe, cough, or talk, or until the victim stops responding.

How to Help a Choking Infant

When an infant is choking and suddenly cannot breathe or make any sounds, you must act quickly to help get the object out by using back slaps and chest thrusts.

Follow these steps to relieve choking in an infant:

Step	Action
1	Hold the infant facedown on your forearm. Support the infant's head and jaw with your hand. Sit or kneel and rest your arm on your lap or thigh.
2	Give up to 5 back slaps with the heel of your free hand between the infant's shoulder blades (Figure 5).
3	If the object does not come out after 5 back slaps, turn the infant onto his back. Move or open the clothes from the front of the chest only if you can do so quickly. You can push on the chest through clothes if you need to.
4	Give up to 5 chest thrusts using 2 fingers of your free hand to push on the breastbone (Figure 6). • Support the head and neck. • Hold the infant with one hand and arm, resting your arm on your lap or thigh.
5	Alternate giving 5 back slaps and 5 chest thrusts until the object comes out and the infant can breathe, cough, or cry, or until the infant stops responding.

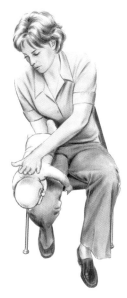

Figure 5. Give up to 5 back slaps with the heel of your hand.

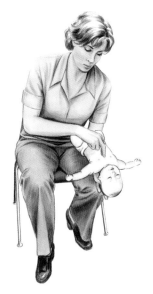

Figure 6. Give up to 5 chest thrusts.

When to Stop Back Slaps and Chest Thrusts

Stop back slaps and chest thrusts if

- The object comes out
- The infant begins to breathe, cough, or cry
- The infant stops responding

Actions for a Choking Infant Who Stops Responding

If you cannot remove the object, the infant will stop responding. When the infant stops responding, follow these steps:

Step	Action
1	Yell for help. If someone comes, send that person to phone your emergency response number (or 911).
2	Place the infant on a firm, flat surface. If possible, place the infant on a surface above the ground, such as a table. This makes it easier to give CPR to the infant.
3	Start the steps of CPR if you know how. Remember to look in the infant's mouth and remove any object you see before giving breaths. If you don't know CPR, phone your emergency response number (or 911) and the dispatcher can tell you what to do.

Allergic Reactions

Many allergic reactions are mild, but you should remember that a mild allergic reaction can become a bad allergic reaction within minutes.

Signs of Mild and Bad Allergic Reactions

The following table shows signs of mild and bad allergic reactions:

Mild Allergic Reaction	Bad Allergic Reaction
• A stuffy nose, sneezing, and itching around the eyes • Itching of the skin • Raised, red rash on the skin (hives)	• Trouble breathing • Swelling of the tongue and face • Fainting

Actions for Bad Allergic Reactions

A bad allergic reaction can be life-threatening and is an emergency. Follow these steps if you see signs of a *bad* allergic reaction:

Step	Action
1	Make sure the scene is safe.
2	Phone or send someone to phone your emergency response number (or 911) and get the first aid kit.
3	If the child is showing signs of a bad allergic reaction and has an epinephrine pen, ask the child to use it. (See the following section for instructions on how to use an epinephrine pen.)
4	If the child stops responding, start the steps of CPR if you know how. If you don't know how, the dispatcher can tell you what to do.
5	If possible, save a sample of what caused the reaction. This may be helpful if this is the child's first allergic reaction.

How to Use an Epinephrine Pen

The epinephrine injection is given in the side of the thigh. There are 2 doses of epinephrine pens, one for adults and one for children. Make sure you have the epinephrine pen prescribed for that child.

Follow these steps to use an epinephrine pen:

Step	Action
1	Get the prescribed epinephrine pen.
2	Take off the safety cap. Follow the instructions printed on the package.
3	Hold the epinephrine pen in your fist without touching either end because the needle comes out of one end.
4	Press the tip of the pen hard against the side of the child's thigh, about halfway between the hip and knee. You can give the epinephrine pen directly to the skin or through clothing (Figure 7).
5	Hold the epinephrine pen in place for several seconds. Some of the medicine will remain in the pen after you use it.
6	Rub the injection spot for several seconds.

(continued)

Step	Action
7	After using the epinephrine pen, give it to the EMS rescuers for proper disposal.
8	Write down the time of the injection. This information may be important for the trained help who cares for the child.
9	Stay with the child until trained help arrives and takes over.

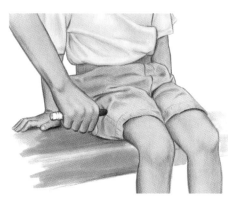

Figure 7. You can give the epinephrine pen directly to the skin or through clothing.

Seizures

Some Causes of Seizures

A medical condition called epilepsy often causes seizures. But *not all* seizures are due to epilepsy. Seizures can also be caused by

- Head injury
- Low blood sugar
- Heat-related emergency
- Poisons
- Fever

Signs of a Seizure

During some types of seizures, the child may

- Lose muscle control
- Fall to the ground
- Have jerking movements of the arms and legs and sometimes other parts of the body
- Stop responding

Actions for a Seizure

Most seizures stop within a few minutes. Follow these steps if you suspect a child is having a seizure:

Step	Action
1	Protect the child from harm by • Moving furniture or other objects out of the child's way • Placing a pad or towel under the child's head
2	Phone or send someone to phone your emergency response number (or 911) if • This is the child's first seizure • You are unsure whether the child has had a seizure before • Your first aid action plan for this child says to do so
3	After the seizure, check to see if the child is breathing. If the child does not respond, start the steps of CPR if you know how. If you don't know how, the dispatcher can tell you what to do.
4	If you do not think that the child has a head, neck, or spine injury, roll the child to his side.
5	Stay with the child until he starts responding.
6	If you have phoned your emergency response number (or 911), stay with the child until trained help arrives and takes over.

After a seizure it is not unusual for the child to be confused or fall asleep.

Shock

Shock

In children, shock is most often present if the child

■ Loses a lot of blood that you can see or that you can't see

■ Has a bad allergic reaction

■ Has lost fluid, such as with vomiting or diarrhea

Signs of Shock

A child in shock may

■ Feel weak, faint, or dizzy

■ Have pale or grayish skin

■ Act restless, stressed, or confused

■ Be cold and clammy to the touch

Actions for Shock

Follow these steps when giving first aid to a child showing signs of shock:

Step	Action
1	Make sure the scene is safe for you and the child.
2	Phone or send someone to phone your emergency response number (or 911) and get the first aid kit.
3	Help the child lie on her back.
4	If there is no leg injury or pain, raise the child's legs just above the level of the child's heart (Figure 8).
5	Use pressure to stop bleeding that you can see.
6	Cover the child to keep the child warm.

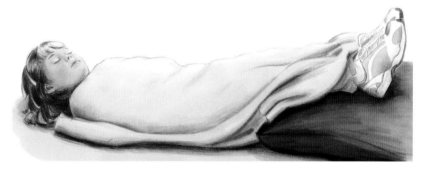

Figure 8. Raise the child's legs just above the level of the heart and cover with a blanket.

Injury Emergencies

Bleeding You Can See

Bleeding You Can See

Bleeding is one of the most frightening emergencies. But many cuts are small and you can easily stop the bleeding. When a large blood vessel is cut or torn, the child can lose a large amount of blood within minutes. That's why you have to act fast.

Actions for Bleeding You Can See

Take the following actions to stop bleeding that you can see:

Step	Action
1	Make sure that the scene is safe for you and the child.
2	Send someone to get the first aid kit.
3	Put firm pressure on the dressing over the bleeding area with the flat part of your fingers or the palm of your hand.
4	If the bleeding does not stop, do not remove the dressing. Add a second dressing and press harder.
5	Check for signs of shock.
6	Phone or send someone to phone your emergency response number (or 911) if • There is a lot of bleeding • You cannot stop the bleeding • You see signs of shock • The injury is from a fall and you suspect a head, neck, or spine injury • You are not sure what to do

Actions for Bleeding From the Nose

Follow these steps when giving first aid to a child with a nosebleed:

Step	Action
1	Make sure the scene is safe for you and the child.
2	Send someone to get the first aid kit.
3	Press both sides of the child's nose while the child sits and leans *forward* (Figure 9).
4	Place constant pressure on both sides of the nose for a few minutes until the bleeding stops.
5	If bleeding continues, press harder.
6	Phone or send someone to phone your emergency response number (or 911) if • You can't stop the bleeding in about 15 minutes • The bleeding is heavy, such as gushing blood • The child has trouble breathing

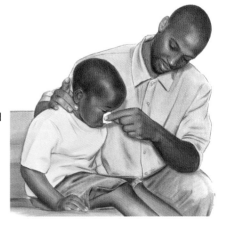

Figure 9. Press both sides of the child's nose while the child sits and leans forward

---

Do Not

When trying to stop a nosebleed

- *Do not* ask the child to lean his head back.
- *Do not* use an icepack on the nose or forehead.
- *Do not* press on the bridge of the nose between the eyes (the upper bony part of the nose).

Bleeding From the Mouth

Like other bleeding you can see, you can usually stop bleeding from the mouth with pressure. But bleeding from the mouth can be serious if blood or broken teeth block the airway and cause breathing problems or if you can't reach the bleeding area.

Actions for Bleeding From the Mouth

Follow these steps when giving first aid to a child with bleeding from the mouth:

Step	Action
1	Make sure the scene is safe for you and the child.
2	Send someone to get the first aid kit.
3	If the bleeding is from the tongue, lip, or cheek or another area you can easily reach, press the bleeding area with a sterile gauze or clean cloth.
4	If bleeding is deep in the mouth and you can't reach it easily, roll the child to his side.
5	Look for signs of shock.
6	Check the child's breathing. Be ready to start the steps of CPR if needed and if you know how.
7	Phone or send someone to phone your emergency response number (or 911) if • You can't stop the bleeding • The child has trouble breathing

Tooth Injuries

Children with a mouth injury may have broken, loose, or knocked-out teeth. This can be a choking hazard, especially for young children.

Actions for Tooth Injuries

Follow these steps when giving first aid to a child with a tooth injury:

Step	Action
1	Make sure the scene is safe for you and the child.
2	Send someone to get the first aid kit.
3	Check the child's mouth for any missing teeth, loose teeth, or parts of teeth.
4	If a tooth is loose, have the child bite down on a piece of gauze to keep the tooth in place and call the child's dentist.
5	If a tooth is chipped, gently clean the injured area and call the child's dentist.
6	If the child lost a permanent tooth, rinse the tooth in water, put the tooth in a cup of milk, and immediately take the child and tooth to a dentist or emergency department.

(continued)

Step	Action
7	Apply pressure with gauze to stop any bleeding at the empty tooth socket.
8	Talk with a dentist if a child's tooth changes color after an injury.

Do Not

- *Do not* hold the tooth by the root. Hold the tooth only by the crown (the part of the tooth that does not go into the gums).
- *Do not* try to reinsert the tooth.

Injuries From Puncturing Objects

An object such as a knife or sharp stick can cause an injury that punctures the skin. It is important not to remove the object. Leave it in place until trained help can treat the injury.

Actions for Injuries From Puncturing Objects

Follow these steps when giving first aid to a child with an injury from a puncturing object:

Step	Action
1	Make sure the scene is safe for you and the child.
2	Phone or send someone to phone your emergency response number (or 911) and get the first aid kit.
3	Stop any bleeding you can see.
4	Try to keep the child from moving.
5	Check for signs of shock.

Bleeding You Can't See

Bleeding You Can't See

A strong hit to the chest or belly or a fall can cause injury and bleeding inside the body. You may not see signs of this bleeding on the outside of the body at all, or you may see a bruise on the skin over the injured part of the body. An injury inside the body may be minor or severe.

When to Suspect Bleeding You Can't See

Suspect bleeding inside the body if a child has

- An injury from a car crash, a pedestrian injury, or a fall from a height
- Pain in the chest or belly after an injury
- Shortness of breath after an injury
- Coughed-up or vomited blood after an injury
- Signs of shock without bleeding that you can see

Actions for Bleeding You Can't See

Follow these steps when giving first aid to a child who may have bleeding you can't see:

Step	Action
1	Make sure the scene is safe for you and the child.
2	Phone or send someone to phone your emergency response number (or 911) and get the first aid kit.
3	Gently try to keep the child still and lying down.
4	Check for signs of shock.
5	If the child stops responding, start the steps of CPR if you know how. If you don't know how, the dispatcher can tell you what to do.

Head Injuries

Head Injury

You should suspect that the child has a head injury if the child

- Fell from a height
- Was hit in the head
- Was injured while diving
- Was electrocuted
- Was involved in a car crash
- Was riding a bicycle or motorbike, was involved in a crash, and has no helmet or a broken helmet

FYI: Falling From a Height

If a child falls from a height greater than the child's height, you should think the child might have a head, neck, or spine injury.

Important: Shaken Baby Syndrome

Shaking a baby can seriously injure a baby. It might even kill the baby. Be sure to handle a baby carefully to protect him or her from injury.

Signs of Head Injury

You should suspect that a child has a head injury if after an injury the child

- Does not respond or only moves or moans and groans
- Is sleepy or confused
- Vomits
- Complains of a headache
- Has trouble seeing
- Has trouble walking or moving any part of the body
- Has a seizure

Actions for Head Injuries

Follow these steps when giving first aid to a child with a possible head injury:

Step	Action
1	Make sure the scene is safe for you and the child.
2	Phone or send someone to phone your emergency response number (or 911) and get the first aid kit.
3	Hold the head and neck so that the head and neck do not move, bend, or twist.
4	Turn or move the child only if • The child is in danger • You need to do so to check breathing or open the child's airway • The child is vomiting
5	If the child does not respond, start the steps of CPR if you know how. If you don't know how, the dispatcher can tell you what to do.

Step	Action
6	If you must turn the child, be sure to roll the child while you support the child's head, neck, and body in a straight line so that they do not twist, bend, or turn in any direction (Figure 10). You will need 2 people to do this.
7	If the child responds and is vomiting, roll the child onto his side.

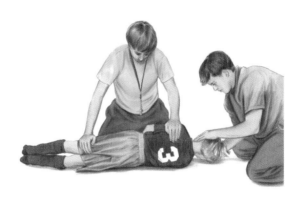

Figure 10. Support the head, neck, and body in a straight line so that they do not twist, bend or turn in any direction.

Broken Bones, Sprains, and Bruises

Broken Bones, Sprains, and Bruises

Broken bones, sprains, and bruises are common in children. Without an x-ray, it may be impossible to tell whether a bone is broken. But you will perform the same actions even if you don't know whether the bone is actually broken.

Bruises

A child may get a bruise if he is hit or runs into a hard object. Bruises happen when blood collects under the skin. They can appear as red or black-and-blue marks. You can reduce swelling by putting an ice bag wrapped in a towel on the bruise.

Actions for Broken Bones and Sprains

Follow these steps when giving first aid to a child with a possible broken bone or sprain:

Step	Action
1	Make sure the scene is safe for you and the child.
2	Send someone to get the first aid kit. If you are alone, go get the first aid kit.
3	Check for signs of shock.
4	Don't try to straighten any injured part that is bent.
5	Cover any open wound with a clean dressing.
6	Put a plastic bag filled with ice on the injured area with a towel between the ice bag and the skin for up to 20 minutes (Figure 11).
7	Raise the hurt body part if doing so does not cause the child more pain.
8	Phone or send someone to phone your emergency response number (or 911) if • There is a large open wound • The injured part is oddly bent • You're not sure what to do
9	If it hurts, the child should try not to use that body part until checked by a healthcare provider.

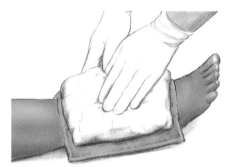

Figure 11. Put ice on an injured area with a towel between the ice bag and skin.

Burns and Electrocution

Overview   Burns are injuries caused by contact with heat, electricity, or chemicals.

Actions for   Follow these steps to give first aid to a child with a small burn:
Small Burns

Step	Action
1	Make sure the scene is safe for you and the child.
2	Send someone to get the first aid kit. If you are alone, go get the first aid kit.
3	If the burn area is small, cool it immediately with cold, but not ice cold, water.
4	You may cover the burn with a dry, nonstick sterile or clean dressing.
5	Phone or send someone to phone your emergency response number (or 911) if • There is a fire • The child has a large burn • You are not sure what to do
6	Contact the child's healthcare provider for any burn.

Actions for Large Burns

Follow these steps to give first aid to a child with a large burn:

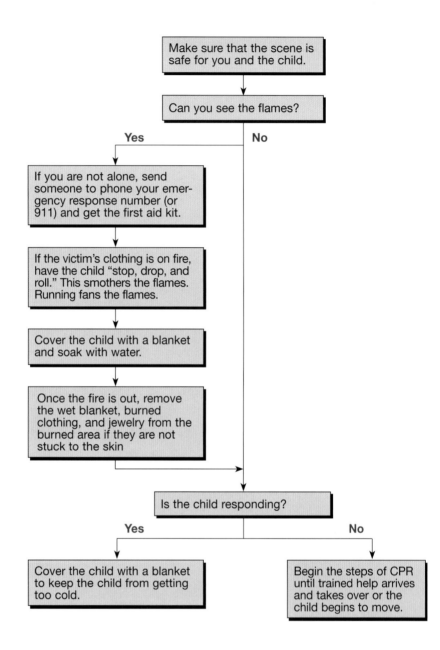

Make sure that the scene is safe for you and the child.

Can you see the flames?

Yes — No

Yes:

If you are not alone, send someone to phone your emergency response number (or 911) and get the first aid kit.

If the victim's clothing is on fire, have the child "stop, drop, and roll." This smothers the flames. Running fans the flames.

Cover the child with a blanket and soak with water.

Once the fire is out, remove the wet blanket, burned clothing, and jewelry from the burned area if they are not stuck to the skin

Is the child responding?

Yes — No

Yes: Cover the child with a blanket to keep the child from getting too cold.

No: Begin the steps of CPR until trained help arrives and takes over or the child begins to move.

Contact the child's healthcare provider for any burn.

Electrical Injury

Electricity can cause burns on the skin and injure organs inside the body.

If electricity enters the body, it can cause severe damage. You may see marks or wounds where the electricity has entered and left the body. These marks may seem very small, but you can't tell from the outside of the body how much damage there is inside the body!

Actions for Electrical Injury

Follow these steps to give first aid to a child with an electrical injury:

Step	Action
1	Make sure the scene is safe for you and the child. Do not touch the child as long as the child is in contact with the power source.
2	Phone or send someone to phone your emergency response number (or 911) and get an AED if one is available.
3	When it is safe to touch the child, check for a response. If the child does not respond or stops responding, start the steps of CPR and use the AED if available. If you don't know how, the dispatcher can tell you what to do.
4	Check for signs of shock.
5	A healthcare provider should check all children who have an electrical injury.

Remember: Although there are many creams and ointments available for burns, it is important that you talk with the child's healthcare provider before using one.

Eye Injuries

Signs of Eye Injuries

Eye injuries may occur with a

- Direct hit or punch in the eye or to the side of the head
- Ball or other object that directly hits the eye
- High-speed object that strikes the eye, such as a BB gun pellet
- Stick or other sharp object that punctures the eye
- Small object in the eye, such as a piece of dirt, an eyelash, a piece of sand, or pollen
- Chemical that splashes in the eye

Signs of eye injury include

- Pain
- Trouble seeing
- Bruising
- Bleeding
- Redness, swelling

Actions for Eye Injuries

Follow these steps for eye injuries:

Step	Action
1	Make sure the scene is safe for you and the child.
2	Send someone to get you the first aid kit. If you are alone, go get the first aid kit.
3	If a child is hit hard in the eye or if an object punctures the eye, seek emergency help. For a puncture, cover the eye with a clean, dry dressing. Tell the child to keep both eyes closed until trained help arrives and takes over.

4	If the eye is not punctured and a chemical or small irritant (such as eyelashes or sand) is in the eye, use running water from a faucet to rinse the irritant from the eye. Make sure the eye with the irritant is the lower eye as you rinse the eye (Figure 12). Make sure you do not rinse the irritant into the unaffected eye.
5	If the object does not come out, or if the child complains about extreme pain, phone the child's healthcare provider. Tell the child to keep both eyes closed until trained help arrives and takes over.

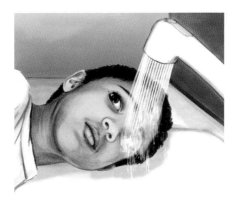

Figure 12. Rinse the eye with running water. Make sure the eye with the irritant is the lower eye.

Environmental Emergencies

Bites and Stings

Animal and Human Bites

Young, preschool-aged children sometimes bite each other. Some young children will bite others to show their feelings. Most children stop biting when they grow older.

Animal bites are less common and can often be prevented. But when they do happen, animal bites can be serious.

Although many bites are minor, some may break the skin. Both animal and human mouths have many germs. When a bite breaks the skin, the wound can bleed and may become infected from the germs in the child's or animal's mouth. Bites that do not break the skin usually are not serious.

Actions for Animal and Human Bites

Follow these steps to give first aid to a child with an animal or a human bite:

Step	Action
1	Make sure the scene is safe for you and the child.
2	Stay away from any animal that is acting strangely. An animal with rabies can bite again.
3	For animal bites, phone or send someone to phone your emergency response number (or 911) and get the first aid kit.
4	Clean the child's wound with running water (and soap if available).
5	Stop any bleeding with pressure.
6	Report all wild animal bites to the police or an animal control officer. Describe • The animal • How the bite happened • The location of the animal when last seen
7	For bites that break the skin, call the child's healthcare provider because the child might need medicine to treat the bite.
8	If there is a bruise or swelling, place an ice bag wrapped in a towel on the bite for up to 20 minutes.

Insect, Bee, and Spider Bites and Stings

Usually insect, bee, and spider bites and stings cause only mild pain, itching, and swelling at the bite.

Some insect bites can be serious and even fatal if

- ■ The child has a bad allergic reaction to the bite or sting
- ■ Poison (venom) is injected into the child (for example, a black widow spider or brown recluse spider)

Actions for Insect, Bee, and Spider Bites and Stings

Follow these steps to give first aid to a child with an insect, bee, or spider bite or sting:

Step	Action
1	Make sure the scene is safe for you and the child.
2	Phone or send someone to phone your emergency response number (or 911) and get the first aid kit if • The child has signs of a bad allergic reaction (see "Actions for Bad Allergic Reactions" on page 18) • The child tells you that she has had a bad allergic reaction to insect bites or stings before
3	If a bee stung the child • Look for the stinger. Bees are the only insects that may leave their stingers behind. • Scrape away the stinger and venom sac using something with a dull edge, such as a credit card.
4	Wash the bite or sting area with running water (and soap if possible).
5	Put an ice bag wrapped in a towel or cloth over the bite or sting area to help reduce swelling.
6	Watch the child for at least 30 minutes for signs of a bad allergic reaction.

Do Not

Do not pull the stinger out with tweezers or your fingers.
Squeezing the venom sac can release more poison (venom).

Poison Emergencies

Poison Control Center Contact Information

The poison control center knows the best way to give first aid for poisonings. The number below will connect you with your nearest poison control center. In many places the poison control hotline can also link the caller directly to the local emergency ambulance dispatch and the nearest hospital's emergency department.

The phone number for the US National Poison Control Center is 800-222-1222. Keep this number close to your phone and in your first aid kit.

FYI: Calling the Poison Control Center

When you phone the poison control center, try to have the following information ready:

- What is the name of the poison? Can you describe it if you cannot name it?
- How much poison did the child touch, breathe, or swallow?
- About how old is the child? About how much does the child weigh?
- When did the poisoning happen?
- How is the child feeling or acting now?

Do Not

During a poison emergency

- *Do not* give the child anything by mouth unless you have been told to do so by trained help or the poison control center. This includes water, milk, syrup of ipecac, and activated charcoal.
- *Do not* rely only on the first aid instructions on the label of the bottle, can, or box.
- *Do not* apply any ointments or lotions to the skin.

Conclusion

Congratulations on taking time to attend this program. Contact the American Heart Association if you want more information on CPR, AEDs, or first aid. You can visit *www. americanheart.org/cpr* or call 877-AHA-4CPR (877-242-4277) to find a class near you.

Even if you don't remember all the first aid steps exactly, it is important for you to try. And always remember to phone your emergency response number (or 911). They can remind you what to do.